Running for Weight Loss

A Running Guide for Safer, Faster Weight Loss

Karina Smith

Table of Contents

INTRODUCTION

Running is one of the greatest exercise styles on the planet. Humans, like most animals have the capacity to run and have used running since prehistoric times to hunt for food, escape predators and in order to survive. With the advance of civilization and technology we have had less need to run but nevertheless still do so at times, without even realizing it.

We run when we're late for the bus. We run after the toddler who is about to cross a busy road. We run to catch up with friends who may have walked on ahead of us. We run because we were designed to run and as we do our body burns calories at a rate far quicker than many other forms of exercise. Even swimming, rowing, cycling and skipping do not burn calories as efficiently as a quick run does.

This book will inform you on ways to use running as an effective fat loss and weight control solution. The advice and tips are ready to use and will give you a running start in achieving your goals for weight control. Often the concept of losing weight is easy to understand but difficult to implement. With the tips and information given here you could be well on your way to a successful weight loss regime. The advice is simple, the implementation easy to execute so if you're ready –let's get running.

Why Should I Run?

There are many benefits to running, the most important of which I will list below. As with any exercise schedule though, you should consult your doctor before embarking on a new exercise program. And remember that running can be strenuous. Take things slowly and build up in small increments to avoid injury.

Whey Running is Great for Weight Loss

Running burns calories fast. It is proven to improve your body's metabolic rate (how active your body is in using energy) and can help you get rid of stubborn fat stores.

Running, especially when you do High Intensity Interval Training(HIIT), has an "after-burn" effect which means that your raised metabolism continues to burn up calories (read: get rid of fat), even after you have stopped running for up to 24 hours!

This phenomenon is known as EPOC (Excess Post Oxygen Consumption) and is limited in most other forms of exercise that do not increase the heart rate significantly.

I'll give you some examples of how to perform HIIT workouts later in this book.

How Running Improves Your Health

Running promotes good cholesterol and boosts the immune system. This aids the body in fighting diseases particularly the onset of diabetes, osteoporosis and high blood pressure. The risk of stroke and even cancers can be significantly reduced with the implementation of a regular running program.

Running is a Very Inexpensive form of Exercise

Compared to many other sports, the outlay for equipment and gear is minimal. Running will only require a good pair of running shoes and some comfortable clothing. It can be performed almost anywhere and does not require expensive gym contracts, the maintenance of equipment or the purchase of highly specialized training programs.

Running Actually Burns More Calories Than any Other Form of Cardio

Minute for minute, a fast run will burn more calories than any static running machine, stair-stepper or cycling machine will do. Running raises the level of fat-burning like no other sport. And it continues to burn fat after you have stopped running!

RUNNING KEEPS YOUR BRAIN SHARP

Running is a stress-relieving activity that affords the mind opportunity to wind down, refocus and clear itself of the troubles and worries of the day. This does wonders for those under stress and provides endorphins which fight depression. Millions of people suffering from these conditions would be much better off if they took up running on a regular basis.

RUNNING STRENGTHENS YOUR JOINTS (WHEN YOU FOLLOW THIS STRATEGY)

It is often thought that running wears out your knees but the opposite is true. Running strengthens the muscles around the knee joints, protecting the all-important cartilage in the knees. More people suffer from knee problems that are overweight or lead sedentary lives. Running can help to get rid of knee and joint pains.

RUNNING HELPS KEEP YOUR BRAIN ALERT

Aging result in a decrease in mental function but running counteracts this degradation in brain function. Running aids memory and keeps the brain alert as your fitness levels increase.

Running Boosts Confidence

The changes and improvements that running will bring are noticeable within two weeks of starting. This is a lot sooner than the results you gain from weight training and many other forms of exercise. Stamina improves and you will see a dip in the scales as your weight begins to drop.

As you begin to feel less breathless and your times improving, it will motivate you to run harder and faster to meet your goals –a winning formula all round.

Taking the 1st Step (Don't Skip This Vital Step)

Before you get your running shoes on and head out onto the roads –Stop! Get a pen and paper. Write down why you want to run. Your motivation is an emotional decision and it is important to voice this decision. Give it some thought…not 'I want to lose 20 pounds' but 'I want to fit into that sexy dress.' Don't write that you want to be fit; you want to be able to run after your kids and not lose your breath. You want bragging rights.

Get creative with your reasons and connect your thoughts to the deepest desires within you. The more your desire for running is connected to things you love and want for yourself, the more you will be motivated to keep up with your program in order to reach your goals. On those days when you don't feel like running and you're just not in the mood, your motivation is what will get you out of bed and into those running shoes.

SETTING ACHIEVABLE GOALS

Are you a regular New Year's resolution breaker? You probably hate the idea of sitting goals. But don't lose heart because you haven't been able to keep those resolutions all these years. Most unmet resolutions are the result of unrealistic goal setting.

This guide will help you set achievable goals by raising your targets in small increments. You're not going to aim to be an Olympic runner within the next two months.

Step one in getting yourself goal-oriented is to get yourself a journal. Take time to get yourself into the routine of tracking your progress and celebrating your victories.

The realistic goals you should be thinking about and setting can look as follows:

- I will run 5 times a week for half an hour

- I will aim to eat 500 less calories a day than my current intake.
- I will cut out sodas, sweet treats and cake for 6 days a week.
- I will push myself harder during a run and take less breaks.
- I will aim to reduce my running times by 20 seconds a week.

These goals are measureable, achievable and realistic. You can achieve them with some will power and in doing so you will boost your confidence. You have the ability to control these targets and meet them. Doing so will keep you motivated to the end goal of a desired weight.

KEEPING A RUNNING JOURNAL

The first thing to journal is your weight. Do this once a week. Don't take a daily reading as your weight varies from day to day. Also watching your weight every day can really impact your motivation negatively when you don't see a change.

Don't be discouraged if your weight loss plateaus. This is typical during any weight loss program. The record of your weight is a guide only and usually indicates that you will need to change things in your running schedule. A break in training may be needed or a change in diet plan could be called for.

The second step in your journaling is to record 3 daily entries:
- Your total food intake (including that slice of cake at the office birthday.)
- Your training program (route, time taken, distance)
- How you felt on the run (Was it easy? Tough? Did you have pain?)
-

Alongside taking your initial weight reading, you may want to do a body fat composition analysis. This can be done with a doctor or at your local gym with a personal trainer. Many trainers offer free initial assessments with no obligation to join the gym.

Alternatively you can just do some measurements with a tape measure.

Take the following readings:
- Around your biceps
- Around the middle of your thigh
- Your belly
- Round your hips
- Your butt

Weight itself is not an entirely useful reading as your mass may increase if you build muscle. And muscle is denser than fat, meaning that while you will be looking leaner you may actually increase your mass.

That is why I always suggest to keep track of your measurements rather than just your weight. Typically when you belly measurement is coming down you overall body fat is coming down with it. So it gives you a much more accurate gauge of your progress than checking your weight alone.

Trust me on this...and don't become a junky of checking your scale. Resist the urge.

There are a number of truly helpful apps for iPad and other tablets that will assist you in keeping accurate records of your eating habits and running schedule so check the app store on your phone or tablet for find one that fits your style.

How Much Weight Loss Should You Expect?

So many infomercials promise amazing weight loss results. The reality is that such quick weight loss isn't realistically achievable without exercise and can be detrimental to your health. Many supplements can give the illusion of having lost weight but they only serve to cause water loss and effectively dehydrate the body – again an unhealthy alternative.

A realistic weight loss of 1-2 pounds per week will mean 15 weeks of work to lose 15-30 pounds. It took you some time to gain the week, it is to be expected that it will take time to lose it again.

Consistency is the key with weight loss and improving your running times

Nutrition

Nutrition is a HUGE part of losing weight. Don't be fooled by these advertisements stating weight loss is all about "green coffee beans", "Acai berries", or any other magical pill. Sure those things have their place but truth be told 90% of your nutrition results come from what you eat every day....NOT a magical pill.

SHOULD I BE COUNTING CALORIES?

This really depends on the weight loss goals you have. Don't obsess over it. If you are simply wanting to let go of some excess body fat, a thorough calorie count may be overkill. Just remain consistent in your efforts to eat a bit less and lose the weight gradually.

If however your aim is to get a set of ripped abs and you need to maintain a body fat ratio of less than 10% then a calorie count is mandatory.

If you don't know how many calories you currently eating then I would also suggest that you track your food for a few days just to see where you are starting out. I find that most of my clients have no idea how many calories they are actually eating!

So where does one begin?

For starters you will need to know what calorie count is conducive for your body to begin losing weight.

A great app for tracking your calories is called **MY FITNESS PAL**. If you don't have a smart phone or a tablet you can sign up on your computer as well.

I have found that the calorie suggestions that My Fitness Pal suggests are typically pretty good suggestions based on the goals that you set when you sign up.

PROTEINS, CARBS AND FAT

One suggestion I would make though is to alter the "macronutrient" settings from within the "goals".

For a good place to start **set your goals at 40% carbohydrates, 30% protein and 30% fat**.

Being aware of the numbers will assist you in planning a suitable eating plan.

Now that you know how much protein, carbs, and fat your should be eating let's talk about quality of food.

Now I'm a big a big fan of what's called "flexible dieting". Basically what that means is that if you allowed to eat 150 grams of protein on for your goals then you can eat whatever foods that you would like to get in your 150 grams of protein over the course of the day. A word of caution though...quality does matter! So the better quality of protein, carbs and fats you eat the better your results with weight loss (and your overall health) will be. Make sense?

Okay so let's go over what are quality protein, carbs and fats?

Protein
Turkey
Chicken breast
Lean beef
Egg whites
Protein powder
Greek yogurt
Cottage cheese
Fish
Etc...

Carbs
Oatmeal
Sweet potatoes
White potatoes

Brown rice
Quinoa
Vegetables
Ezekiel bread
Etc...

Fats
Nuts
Seeds
Olive oil
Macadamia oil
Avocado
Egg yolks
Etc...
*Note: you will get some fat in your meats as well but if your choosing lean cuts of meat it should be kept to a minimum.

So the more calories you can consume from quality sources of food as I have outlined the better results you will get!

Here are some dieting Do's and Don'ts

DIETING DO's:
- Calculate your total calorie intake daily
- Eat regular small meals throughout the day coupled with good intakes of water
- Check the labeling of foods for calorie counts
- Exercise regularly

DIETING DON'TS

- Change your food intake radically –cut amounts in small increments
- Miss meals or starve yourself –your body will only go into starvation mode and store fat
- Replace your old foods with new unfamiliar foods all at once. Gradually eat less of the foods you always used to eat and slowly replace with other healthier alternatives. Your body needs to get used to a new eating plan and won't respond well to a sudden shock eating plan. It's not out with the pizza and in with the broccoli. You're bound to have a rejection reaction from your body.

BEFORE YOU GET STARTED RUNNING

There are some essential things to tick off in preparation for a successful running and weight loss program.

PICKING OUT THE PERFECT RUNNING SHOES

Since this is one of the few, if not only investments that you will make, it is worth spending on the best pair you can afford. Running injuries are nearly always attributed to poor shoes that either don't fit properly or offer decent support.

Since running is an impact sport, it is important that shoes cushion the impact properly. Enlist the help of qualified running shoe specialists at a store that will give you the best advice.

Each person is different and will require a different shoe depending on your arch, your motion mechanics and your foot strike. A flat foot may need shoes with a higher arch for example.

Get the right shoe and sizing for your feet from day one. This will prevent all kinds of injuries.

Here is a great resource called "Shoe Advisor" for finding the perfect running shoe for you:

http://www.runnersworld.com/shoe-finder/shoe-advisor

Also note the day you buy them and keep a record of their mileage (yes, just like you do for your vehicle). You will need to replace them after 400 miles (640km). Don't judge your shoes by their outward appearance. The inner cushioning will have worn out by then and the strain on your knees, risk of shin splints or doing yourself an injury is not worth a few more miles in old shoes.

Preferably if you can afford it, buy two pairs and alternate. The shoes will last longer as the cushioning has a longer period to dry out and decompress. This gets more life out of your shoe.

About halfway through the time of using one pair, buy a new pair and begin to run them in. If you can, also keep a fresh pair as a reference so that you can judge when the older pair needs replacement.

Following this procedure for use will extend the life of your running shoes to the upper limits of a shoe's life of around 400 miles. You will also be able to donate a reasonable looking pair to organizations that collect old pairs of shoes for needy athletes.

The Best Running Clothes For Your body Type

There is a large variety of clothing made for runners. Some prefer tight fitting clothing like ski pants or leggings. Others prefer looser clothing e.g. a baggy T-shirt. Some men prefer running without a shirt. Women will need a sports bra and for both men and women decent sports socks are essential. These need to be made from synthetic materials as they are better at preventing blisters, unlike cotton socks.

Some wonderful new designs are available in clothing made for runners which feature such unique developments as removing excess water from the skin, hence keeping you cooler. The clothing is also designed not to chafe the skin making it more comfortable for the really long runs.

Stopwatches

This is an essential product for tracking ongoing progress. You will want to keep track of things such as how long it takes to run a specific distance. Sometimes you will want to see if you have taken even twenty seconds off your time. Becoming accurate about your distances and timings is essential in developing good tracking habits.

Depending on what you want to track and your budget there are a wide variety of watches.

You can now track things like heart rate, distance and intervals with your watch.

For that reason I like 3 specific brands

1. Polar
2. Nike
3. Garmin

Most of their running watches are equipped with all of the latest features.

Heart rate training can be especially useful for weight loss aspect of training.

If you're going to be training for a distance race, like a 5k, in conjunction with your weight loss training the GPS watches can really be nice!

Again it all depends on what your specific goals are and your budget but shop take some time to shop around and find the right watch for you.

WATER BOTTLES

While not an essential, you may be a runner who gets thirsty on the run and having a water bottle at hand can be a life-saver on a hot day. The plastic BPA bottles are the safest while running.

ANKLE WEIGHTS

These are great for improving stamina once you are fitter. They are comfortable additions to your ankles that force your body to adapt to a more challenging run. You will find them invaluable in creating more stamina and strengthening your body.

ANTI-CHAFE BALM

Chafing can be painful and interrupt your training routine. A good anti-chafe balm will soothe skin that has become irritated and inflamed. This can be gotten from a good sports store or ordered online from Amazon.

You may want to consider other items, including headphones, headbands, heart rate monitors, sunglasses etc. but many of these are simply luxury extras and not necessary for a great run.

BEFORE YOU START RUNNING

Once you have all the equipment organized and you're all set, ready to go take a moment to prepare yourself for the run.

Three essentials before you step out onto the road are:

- Warming Up
- Stretching
- Hydrating

You need to get the blood flowing in your body. A couple of jumping jacks, burpees or similar exercises or even a light round of skipping will get the heart rate up and start pumping the blood through your body.

After your body is feeling a little more energized you will need to do a thorough stretch, focusing especially on the knees, ankles, calves hamstrings and waist. Also do some limbering up of the upper body so as to get mobile.

Around five minutes of stretching should be enough to get your body ready and prepped for running. Lastly you need to remain hydrated for a good running experience. Don't drink large amounts just before a run but ensure that throughout the day you are receiving the correct amounts of water. Sipping throughout the day is recommended and you should carry a water bottle with you wherever you go.

COMMON RUNNING MISTAKES

There are some potential hazards to a successful running program. To avoid injury, here are some pitfalls you should avoid to give yourself the best opportunity for success.

Don't stretch a cold body. A static stretch routine can lead to injury. Cold stretches lead to a decrease in muscle strength. It is essential to first get your body warm through some active exercises such as skipping or burpees. Getting the heart rate up is essential and then only a mild stretch is needed to prepare you for your run.

Never wear old or worn shoes. That's it –Just don't do it

Keep your expectations real. Take things slow and don't go for too much too soon. A week of running a successful two or three kilometres is better than attempting five kilometres and getting stiff and having to interrupt your running schedule. You are not out to torture yourself on your run.

Don't keep to the same route and running tempo throughout. You should vary your heart rate by putting in some sprints, running up hills and choosing more challenging routes from time to time. Not only is this great for your heart rate, strength and stamina but it will also keep you burning that fat even after you have ended your run.

Not keeping your carb-level up. You need fuel to run and to avoid that slumping feeling from a drop in sugar level you will need a steady flow of energy that should be sourced from healthy carbohydrates.

Watch your stride. Over-striding is caused when your heel is landing past your body's centre of gravity. A smaller stride maintains a better level of energy conservation. Some runners feel they are running faster by making bigger strides but they are using more energy than they need. It also results in a greater chance of getting shin splints.

Not paying attention to your upper body form is a sure-fire way to limit your progress. On the road you will notice all kinds of unusual postures; arms flopping all over the place, odd strides, heads being held at an odd angle and the like. You should be keeping your arms at ninety degrees, at waist level and close to your hip. Your chest should be out and you need to maintain an upright posture, while swinging your arms lightly back and forth as you run. Avoid letting your arms cross your body while you run.

Not resting between runs –this is a common cause of injury and one of the most common errors in a running program. The body needs time to recover from a run and to replenish its glycogen stores. It also stresses your body and causes it to release the hormone known as cortisol. This hormone indirectly leads to weight gain. The rests in between are as important as the runs you do. Remember that great music is made because of the spaces in between the notes.

Don't just be a runner! While running is great exercise, other forms of exercise are also necessary to increase your strength and overall fitness. Interspersing your running schedule with a once-a-week swim or weight training session will help you maintain a better overall body development and it varies things up a bit to keep you interested.

Don't be too tensed up when you run.. It is important to relax your body while you run so as to achieve better performances. Breathe consistently and evenly while you run. Keep your shoulders dropped and don't clench the jaw. You will need to make a conscious effort to relax while running. This will help you focus and stay in the zone while running.

Not drinking enough water. This will result in dehydration, which effectively tires your body out and can even result in lost performance and even heat stroke in extreme circumstances. Electrolyte drinks are also useful from time to time in order to replace lost minerals and salts. Just watch the sugar if you running for weight loss.

RUNNING TECHNIQUES AND TIPS

Running is a natural body activity unlike weight training which requires many adjustments in forms and methods. It is an easy sport to become quite good at doing as long as one adheres to some general basics. It is quite possible to become a good runner just by keeping a regular schedule that is calculated to improve your skills over time.

Naturally you will need to actually go out and run to lose the weight. Just reading this book won't do it for you. When you sweat the fat will drop off you. So here are some considerations for getting the fat to drop off quicker.

SHOULD I RUN ON AN EMPTY STOMACH?

It is a question that has been debated by some. It is definitely recommended and one should run after waking up as this is a time when the body's glycogen stores are low. Since the body needs the glycogen it will convert fat stores into glycogen hence burning fat instead of breaking down muscle.

Two things need to be kept in mind when running on an empty stomach.

Keep the run to within 20 to 30 minutes. Too long will result in a significant drop of energy.

Keep the run at a steady pace. You should be able to maintain a conversation while you are running. So if you are panting and cannot keep up a conversation it is a sign that your pace is too quick.

It is a great tool to get rid of stubborn fat stores and usually best to alternate between days when you have done a high intensity run.

SHOULD I RUN BAREFOOT

Although some people suggest that barefoot running maintains a natural stride that is altered by wearing shoes, it is generally far more beneficial to run with shoes. Shoes provide cushioning against the high impact nature of running. Also one needs to find very safe places to run barefoot and aside from perhaps a treadmill at home, it is generally recommended that shoes are a better option for just about every running surface.

USING TREADMILLS OR TRACKS?

Treadmills can be useful to maintain a steady rate, which can be adjusted as necessary. The lack of scenery can make it a boring run though and when you're out on the tracks or road, you can adjust your pace as necessary. A treadmill can also be useful during inclement weather or if you want to run at night.

Perhaps safety issues are a concern when out on the road.

It really is a matter of preference but there are pros and cons to both.

CALCULATING MAXIMUM HEART RATE (MHR)

Exercising in the so-called MHR zone pushes the body to increase levels of fitness and stamina. You will need a heart rate monitor to do this. The calculation of maximum heart is gotten by deducting your age from 220. So if you are 40 years of age your maximum heart rate is

$$220 - 40 = 180 \text{ beats per minute}$$

Heart rate can be affected by hydration levels, heat and heart size. Don't exercise beyond the point of discomfort. If you are feeling uncomfortable at a higher heart rate, drop your running level down a notch.

HOW DO I BREATHE WHILE RUNNING?

Breathing is the key to a comfortable run. It is also important to help you run   faster and with less fatigue. Here are 4 points for consideration.

Breathe deeply –even if you feel you don't need the amount of air initially.

Breathe with your belly, not your chest. Your diaphragm (which is situated below your chest) is designed to keep you breathing correctly. Use it while you run.

Pace your breaths to your steps e.g. One breath for every three to four steps is great for a slower running pace. If you increase the pace you will need to take in a breath for every two or even one breath per step. Keep your mouth slightly open while breathing so that air can go in through your nose and mouth.

Your breathing should be a natural part of your run. Deep regular breaths will   ease your running and make your lungs function better.

CAN I IMPROVE MY RUNNING SPEED

There is a wonderful method developed by Adam Kessler that shows you how to train in order to improve your running speed. Adam has had 15 years' experience in improving runners' speed. You can find this method at http://www.howtorunfasternow.com/run-faster-method/

How Do I Lose Weight By Running

Well this is the reason you're taking an interest in running. So here are some   steps to get the weight off.

Keep your daily caloric intake at a deficit. It's a simple rule: If you want to lose weight you need to use more calories than you replace.

Alternate your runs by varying running tempo and use rest days. A typical schedule could look as follows:

Running Schedule:

Monday, Wednesday –high intensity cardio
Tuesday, Friday, Saturday –low to moderate intensity (running on empty stomach for 30 min)
Thursday, Saturday – rest days

Running Workouts

As fitness improves do high intensity for 3 or 4 sessions. A typical workout may look as follows:

WEEK 1 Sprint 30 seconds Walk 30 seconds (Do 15 repetitions)
WEEK 2 Sprint 45 seconds Walk 45 seconds (Do 13 repetitions)

WEEK 3 Sprint 60 seconds Walk 60 seconds (Do 10 repetitions)

If you don't complete all the repetitions don't be too concerned, the point is to get you perspiring and panting. You want to be out of breath by the time you are done.

Train hard but be sensible. Over time stamina will improve and weight will drop off. High intensity exercise is demanding on your body and nervous system. That is why you need to alternate it with low intensity.

As your ability increases, you can increase intensity by finding hills to run. Run up the hill and then walk down. This can offer you a great, exhausting strength workout. If you slip up on your calorie intake (and you will) don't beat yourself up over it. If you haven't given it your all in a workout, relax. Bad days are inevitable. What is important is that you keep at it and get back on track.

Charting your success will reveal some dips in the scale but the overall graph should go up as you continue. Don't let the setbacks get you off track.

DEALING WITH INJURIES

Injuries will happen and all runners experience injuries from time to time. Some injuries can be avoided. Check out http://www/.runnersworld.com/health/big-7-body-breakdowns to learn how to avoid some of the more common injuries. While the internet offers vast amounts of information it is always advisable to consult a doctor if you have done yourself an injury.

Never push your body or think of yourself as invincible. Pushing your body through pain can be dangerous. Rest if you are out of breath. Take time to improve –Rome wasn't built in a day.

Many small improvements are better than aiming for a substantial change and causing problems through injury. Stress fractures will take time to heal and interrupt your training schedule.

FINDING MOTIVATION

"I run because long after my footprints fade away, maybe I will have inspired a few to reject the easy path, hit the trails, put one foot in front of the other, and come to the same conclusion I did: I run because it always takes me where I want to go."

— Dean Karnazes, Ultramarathon Man:

Confessions of an All-Night Runner

Habits take 21 days to form, so a good 4 weeks should do it –counting in those rest days. But even long term runners have days when they don't feel like it. The brain begins to make excuses and guilt sets in because you know you should be going for that run.

This is when you need to find the motivation to go for it, despite those feelings. Giving in to the excuses is a sure-fire recipe to losing the good habit you have begun. Some things just need to be kept going in a repetitive manner –bathing, reading, sleeping… and running. Stop weeding a garden and the weeds grow back. Stop running and you're on the slippery path that led to your initial weight gain.

Some tips on staying motivated

- Change your routes, see new things.

- Vary your times, run early morning or even late at night.
- Find a partner to help you stay accountable to your schedule
- Music can help you keep pace and make the run more relaxing
- Challenge yourself by adding weights or increasing intensity
- Always try and beat your personal best (hence the good journaling)
- Get a subscription to a runner's magazine e.g. Running Times to see what other runners do. Great articles will teach you new things, keep you motivated and inspire you to greatness.
- Enter a Fun Run, 10km or 21km depending on your fitness.

Running is a great sport and one which you can take great pride in. To close off here is another quote from Dean Karnazes for your inspiration.

> *"As long as my heart's still in it, I'll keep going. If the passion's there, why stop?...*
> *There'll likely be a point of diminishing returns, a point where my strength will begin to wane. Until then, I'll just keep plodding onward, putting one foot in front of the other to the best of my ability. Smiling the entire time."*

— Dean Karnazes, Ultramarathon Man:
Confessions of an All-Night Runner

I hope you have found great value in reading this book!

My mission is to help over 1 million people to lose weight with running and truly develop a passion for the sport. You can help me in this mission by leaving a 5 star review on Amazon!

Thank you for your support!

Karina Smith

www.ingramcontent.com/pod-product-compliance
Lightning Source LLC
Chambersburg PA
CBHW061936280526
45787CB00004B/1626